# Blessing Your Baby

### By Wendy Shaw

He gives the
barren woman a home,
making her the joyous mother
of children.
Praise the LORD.

Psalm 113:9

# Table of Contents

# A PRE-BORN BABY'S BILL OF RIGHTS

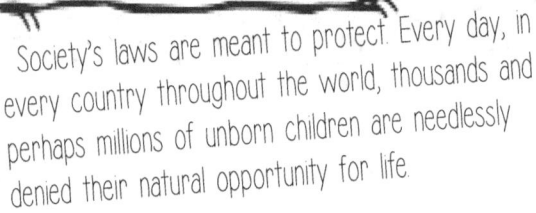

Society's laws are meant to protect. Every day, in every country throughout the world, thousands and perhaps millions of unborn children are needlessly denied their natural opportunity for life.

We hold these truths to be self evident. That every unborn child has:

1 -The right to survive inside the womb.

2 -The right to have adequate nutritional support to develop a healthy mind and body.

3 -The right to be protected from exposure to poisons and toxins and doctors who wish to end their life.

4 -The right to a healthy womb environment free of physical trauma and harmful levels of noise, light, or other excessive stimulation.

5 -The right to be accepted as an individual, alive and aware, and able to feel pain before birth.

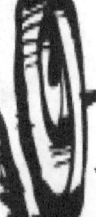

*Adapted from the Fetal Bill of Rights, drafted by Prenatal University.

# Introduction

Every baby, from conception, is special and worthy of protection and love. Each child is unique and wonderfully made. A baby doesn't become a person at birth, it is already living and interacting with its world from deep inside its mother's womb. The prenatal period is the perfect time to begin purposefully showing love to your baby. You don't need to wait until the minute your baby is born to start bonding. There are at least six areas that you can personally bless your baby in, right now! Before its born, you can assure it of a good head start on life.

There are many benefits for everyone when you interact with him/her while he/she is still growing in your womb.

## 3 Benefits of Pre-Birth Bonding:

1- **Parents** who bond with their baby before birth have described their babies as more calm, alert, and happy after birth.

2- **Your baby** will have the advantage of being reassured by familiar voices, sounds, and music that it heard during its time in the womb.

3- **Other family members** will feel more involved with the baby, when they practice bonding beforehand.

Even while snuggled securely inside your womb, your baby is impacted by outside influences. For example, when you are active, healthy, and in a stimulating environment, hormones that stimulate a baby's brain appear to cross the placenta more easily!

As baby grows, each new development provides more opportunities to bond with him/her. You may be surprised just how rapidly he/she is growing after conception!

## What's Happening?

*Week 2*.....Its tiny heart begins to beat.

*Week 5*.....The cerebral cortex is developed. This is the part of the brain that allows this little person to move, think, speak, plan, and create.

*Week 7*.....Baby's head and neck begin to take shape.

*Week 8*.....Its eyes and the ears are beginning to form.

*Week 9*.....He/she can hiccup and react to loud noises.

*Week 12*....Facial expression begin to develop.

*Week 14*....He/she reacts to internal fluctuations in temperature and can differentiate between sweet and bitter tastes.

*Week 16*....Baby can hear.

*Week 18*....Brain development accelerates.

*Week 22*....He/she can hear sounds from outside of the womb and is now sensitive to touch.

*Week 26*.....Your baby experiences the rapid eye movement (REM) sleep of dreams. He/she is more responsive to sound.

*Week 24*....Baby moves in rhythm and may start to show its preferences for particular musical selections.

*Week 34*....Baby can respond differently to mother's, father's and other family member's voices.

## *Between Weeks 38-42, Baby is ready for birth!*

Being intently aware of the environment being created, and having knowledge of how baby is growing, will give your relationship with your little one a special beginning.

This book is divided into 6 Chapters, plus additional resources for family blessings. Each chapter focuses on a key area that you can bless your baby in, and concludes with practical ways to apply that knowledge. These blessings are just a few of the many ways you can develop a special bond with your child. I encourage you to pray and ask the LORD for more specific areas that could directly help your growing family, and you can follow through with your own unique plan.

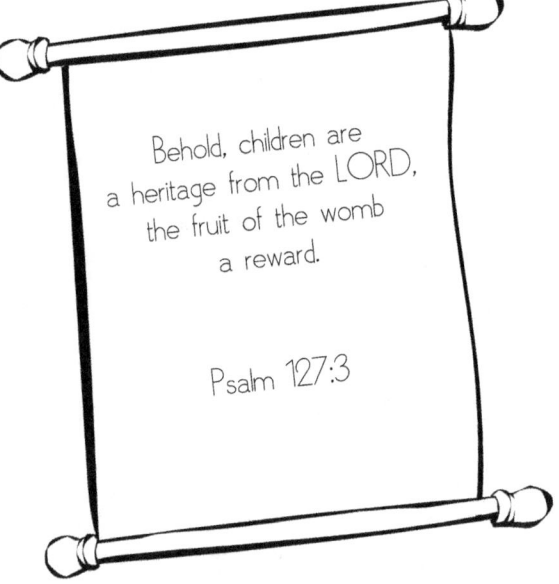

Behold, children are
a heritage from the LORD,
the fruit of the womb
a reward.


Psalm 127:3

## Chapter 1

# Touching

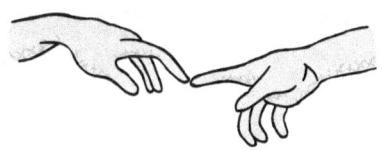

"The Lord called me from the womb,
from the body of my mother he named my name."
Isaiah 49:1

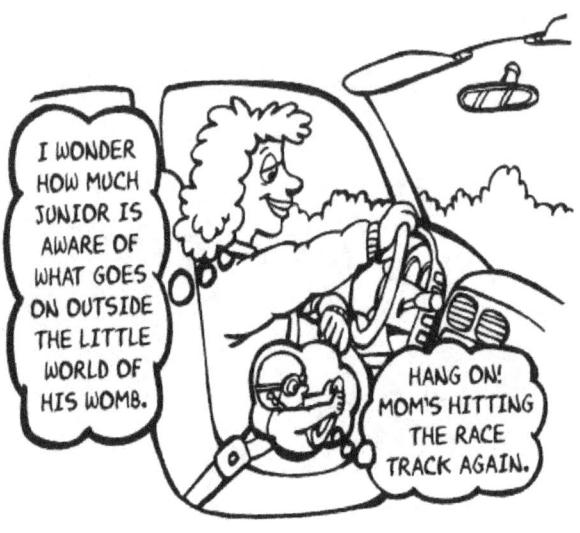

The unborn baby is increasingly aware of sound, light, and touch coming from outside the comfort and protection of its mother's womb.

The experience of being touched has direct and beneficial effects on the growth of the human body as well as on its mind. Research suggests brain chemicals may be released through the act of physical touch. When we touch, we release oxytocin - a bonding chemical. Touching benefits both baby and mom.

It's not too soon to begin. With the advent of sonograms and live-action ultrasound images, neonatologists and nurses are able to see unborn babies react physically to their outside stimuli even at 20 weeks gestation.  (Their sense of touch is so acute that even a single human hair drawn across an unborn child's palm causes the baby to make a fist!) From around 20 weeks your baby will start to feel you touching  through your tummy. Research shows that unborn babies can distinguish between their parents touch, or that of a stranger.

Gentle touching is the best way to convey loving feelings. You may have noticed that you frequently rub, pat or touch your tummy throughout the day.  Once a woman knows she is pregnant, she tends to naturally rest her hands on her tummy.

Touch has a memory.
..........................................
-John Keats, 1821

While moms have a biochemical bond with their babies which connects them to their child before it even leaves the womb, research shows that the same thing can be said for dads, too. Babies respond to their father's touch and their heart rate slows down, or in some cases, speeds up.

Different styles of touching your baby include a gentle pat, rub, soft squeeze, light stroke, tap, or soothing massage on your expanding belly. Press lightly so that it is comfortable for you.

Softly touching or rubbing your belly is a great way to develop early communication with your baby. Rub your belly when your baby moves about and build up an exchange of kicks and rubs.

Don't be surprised if you gently push your tummy and your baby pushes back. There is nothing quite as exciting as feeling your baby respond to your touch for the very first time.

> Make tummy touching a frequent daily exercise.

## *Blessing through Touch*

1- Gently massage your belly. Lay both hands on your stomach and apply light pressure. Use clockwise movements around your belly, then follow by long strokes from top to bottom.

2- Rub anti-stretch mark cream, essential oil (lavender or peppermint) mixed with carrier oil, or plain beneficial coconut oil on tummy.

3- Softly pat your tummy in time to relaxing classical music.

4- As you shower, use the palm of your soapy hand to caress your tummy.

5- Lay your hands on your tummy and pray for your unborn child.

6- Get your husband involved, too. Daddy's slow, gentle strokes can soothe baby and can help you to relax, as well.

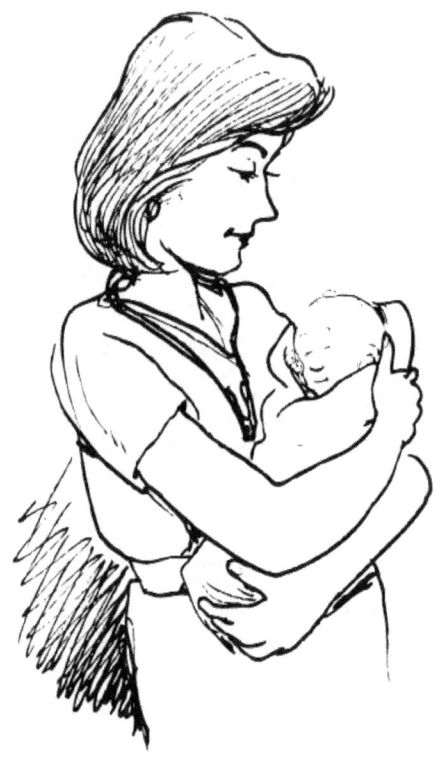

Imprinting begins in the womb.
Soon after a baby is born, he/she may turn its head
in the direction of its mother's voice and is able to
recognize its own mother's unique scent.

# Chapter 2

# Listening

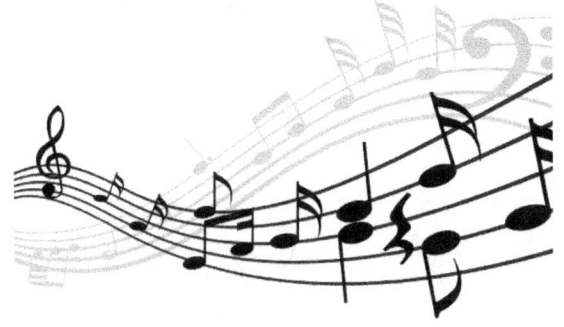

"Make a joyful noise unto the LORD, all the
earth: make a loud noise, and rejoice, and sing praise."
Psalm 98:4

"If music
be the food of love,
play on."

.........................

-William Shakespeare

The best music to a baby's ears is its mother's heartbeat. Many musicologists believe the rhythms and time signature of most musical compositions derive their origins from the human heart rate of about 60 beats per minute. That is why babies are most often soothed by the classical music of Chopin, Mozart and Vivaldi. These composers consistently used tempos that are reminiscent of the human heartbeat.

Researchers say that because classical music has a more complex musical structure and the complexity of it is what primes the brain to solve spatial problems more quickly, classical music may increase learning development and overall well-being. Amazingly - babies as young as 3 months show recognition to higher musical structure and classical music selections they have heard before.

During the first months of pregnancy the baby will not be capable of hearing, but will be able to feel vibrations. The unborn baby will start hear noises outside its Mother's womb starting at the 18th week of pregnancy, so it becomes increasingly important what they are hearing.

Due to the cortex being developed enough to differentiate sounds, a seven month old baby is able to react to different types of music. They seem to kick more in agitation when exposed to rock music and stay calmer when classical music is played. (13)

Research by Andrew Pudewa has shown dramatic effects to our well being by what we listen to. He states in part,

*"Music therapists have shown "New Age" music...decrease(s) mental clarity; "Grunge Rock" increases hostility and decreases relaxation. Most popular, classic rock, alternative, and even a lot of contemporary Christian music is rhythmic dominant. ... Music (with the accent on the off-beat) is not natural, and the... body, which has a rhythmic heartbeat and pulse, perceives this persistent syncopation as an attack, and responds with a release of adrenaline and endorphins.... It creates tension...."(31)*

Statistics have shown that thought and sleep patterns in prenatal development can be influenced by music. Babies are exceptionally receptive to environmental sounds, hence the main goal of prenatal music is to set the stage for an early learning and emotional well being scenario.

Songs with meaningful lyrics, positive, and heartfelt tunes influence our attitudes. When a woman relaxes, that is good for her baby which is an indirect effect of music on her child, as well.

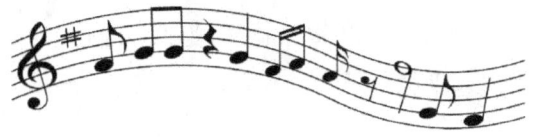

Beneficial music can indirectly calm and focus the mom-to-be throughout her pregnancy.

# ❀ *Blessing through Music*

1- Listen to music from these composers: Bach, Handel, Pachelbel, Vivaldi, Haydn, Mozart, Beethoven. Choose music that relaxes you. Stay away from music that has heavy drumbeats.

2- Listen to sounds of nature like ocean sounds or other nature sounds that soothe you.

3- Purchase a hymnal and sing traditional hymns.

4- Play lullaby songs.

5- Sing happy, uplifting and positive songs. Pay close attention to lyrics. Sometimes the rhythm is catchy, but the words aren't positive.

6- Sing, dance and play music as a family, during and after pregnancy. Your child will recognize these familiar sounds after its born.

## Chapter 3

# Speaking

"A soft answer turns away wrath,
but a harsh word stirs up anger."
Proverbs 15:1.

"Eloquent speech
is not from lip to ear, but rather
from heart to heart."
........................
-William Jennings Bryan

While you learn about your baby, your baby is also learning about you. Your womb is not a silent place. Researchers listened through a hydrophone into the womb of a pregnant woman and picked up many different sounds. These sounds include the whooshing of blood in the vessels, the gurgling and rumbling of the stomach and intestines, and the tones of mother's voice filtered through her tissues, bones, and fluid. These womb sounds stay imprinted on the baby's mind!

By the time baby is born he/she is already familiar with your voice and can distinguish between your voice and that of a stranger. The mother's voice seems to have an impact on her baby. The baby's heart rate slows when the mother is speaking, suggesting that the baby hears and recognizes the familiar sound and is calmed by it. (5) Other Studies indicate that babies attuned to their mother's voices react with an accelerated heartbeat. The infant also responds to a familiar story.(1) Since the baby remembers and recognizes attributes of speech, speaking life and love to it will greatly benefit your growing baby.

# Language

Studies also indicate that whatever a child hears in the womb, he will more easily understand after he is born.

Start communicating with your baby as if he or she is already present with you, by talking, singing or even humming to your baby. This will help him/her begin to recognize your language formations. (20) When a science team recorded and analyzed the cries of 60 healthy newborns, 30 born into French-speaking families and 30 born into German-speaking families, their analysis revealed clear differences in the shape of the newborns' cry melodies, based on their mother tongue. (17) They are responding and developing to what they hear, already! This was the case with John the Baptist, who leaped in his mother's womb when he heard the voice of Mary (see Luke 1:44).

---

Let your speech encourage and edify
the people in your life. Spend time with those who
also practice using their speech wisely.

---

Your voice is very important to your child. A baby will turn its head to the direction of its mother's voice after birth. Even when babies cannot understand actual words, they do react to the tone of voice. Soothing tones calm babies and angry ones upset them. (10)

The Bible says that the power of life and death reside in our tongue. We can either tear someone down, or build them up, by the words we choose to use. Hearing uplifting words, positive affirmations, and soft voices can edify and encourage anyone. Making an effort to speak loving words to your baby can communicate to him/her their valuableness.

"Kindness
is the language which the deaf
can hear and the blind can see."
........................

~Mark Twain

# 20 Positive Phrases to Speak to Baby

1- I love and cherish you.

2- I am so glad you were created.

3- You are very special.

4- May your life be a blessing to many.

5- I am completely happy to be pregnant with you.

6- I love to feel, and watch, you move around.

7- I enjoy being part of your growing process.

8- May God always bless you.

9- You are a treasure.

10- I love that you are a part of my life.

11- I enjoy having you grow inside of me.

12- You are worth any challenge.

13- Good morning (good night), my love.

14- You are precious to me!

15- I look forward to meeting you.

16- I am honored to be your mother.

17- I am thankful for your life.

18- You are a valuable gift to me.

19- Your birth will be a wonderful day.

20- I've never met you, but I love you, already

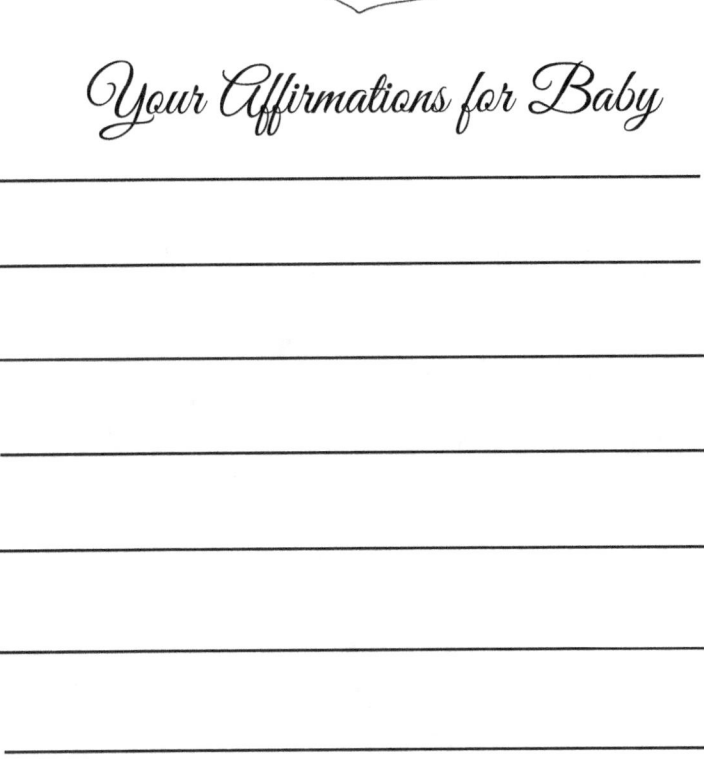

## Your Affirmations for Baby

_____

_____

_____

_____

_____

_____

_____

*Finally, brethren, whatsoever things are true,
whatsoever things are honest, whatsoever things are just, whatsoever things
are pure, whatsoever things are lovely, whatsoever things are of good report;
if there be any virtue, and if there be any praise, think on these things.*

*Philippians 4:8*

# ❀ *Blessing through Speech*

1- Talk out loud about the little activities in your daily life. Share your experiences with your baby no matter how ordinary they may seem to you.

2- Tell your baby you love him/her.

3- Speak positive and comforting words.

4- Pray aloud for the emotional, mental, physical, and spiritual well-being of your child.

5- Treat your baby as a conscious being. Speak kindly and respectfully to him/her.

6- Sing songs or read poems to your baby.

# Chapter 4

# Resting

"*It is in vain that you rise up early and go late to rest,
eating the bread of anxious toil;
for he gives to his beloved sleep.*"
Psalm 127:2

"Every day may not be good,
but there's something good in every day."

..........................

Author Unknown

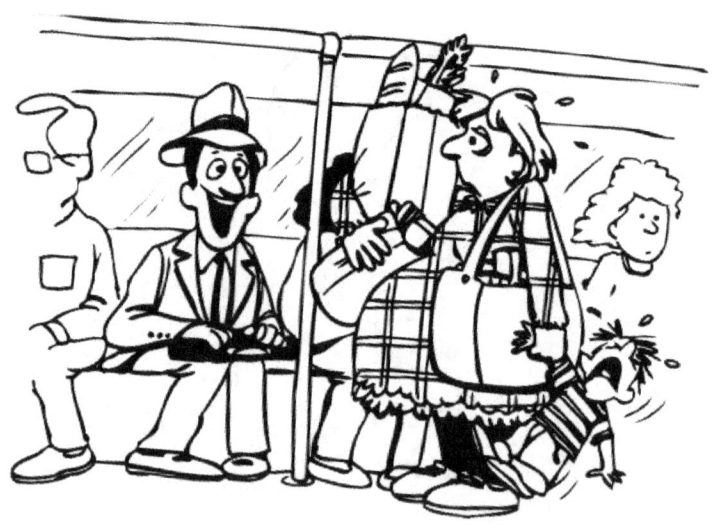

Stress vs. Rest
There are always 2 choices in responding to challenges: Positively or negatively.
Having a sense of humor can help reduce stress.

The feelings and attitudes of the mother are major factors in the baby's health and well being. The relationship between parental attitudes and the infant begin at conception because the baby in the uterus directly shares the mother's emotions at a physiological level.

As early as in the womb, maternal stress has a direct impact on the formation of her baby's personality. Since baby is at a fragile and fertile state of development, be careful about the kind of environment and influences that are created for him/her and you. (21)

Relaxed pleasure states in the expectant mother result in an optimal uterine environment for the baby. Newer studies suggest that babies may hear and feel more than we realize, so when the mother is happy, baby is too! Likewise, when mother is anxious, so is her baby.

*When Mom is stressed, both her and baby react physically.*

**Immune response.** Increased stress is associated with decreased immune system response.

**Hormones.** The hormones a mother puts out in response to stress also appear critical. If a thought or perception is stressful, the mother's pituitary gland secretes a hormone called ACTH which causes her adrenal gland to release other hormones—cortisone and adrenaline-like substances. All of these substances actually bathe the early embryo and later cross the placental barrier and enter the blood stream of the unborn baby.

Highly pressured mothers-to-be tend to have more active pre born babies-- and more irritable infants. "The most stressed are working pregnant women," says researcher DiPietro. It was further demonstrated that mothers who underwent severe emotional stress during pregnancy often had infants who were irritable, hyperactive, and colicky. Other researchers found that such infants tended to be restless and cried a lot.

**Nutrition.** Studies show that anxiety decreases a pregnant woman's ability to absorb nourishment. A mother can fail to retain up to twice as much nitrogen, phosphorus, and calcium as the baby needs. (9)

**Baby's emotions.** There is some connection between a mother's thoughts and her unborn child especially from six months onwards. The mother's emotions result from her thoughts and perceptions which activate both, a part of the mother's nervous system called the autonomic nervous system, and a part of the brain called the hypothalamus. The nervous system and the hypothalamus then affect the tension of the muscle and the output of certain glands. A pre born baby that age can share mother's emotions because of the hormones that cross the placenta.

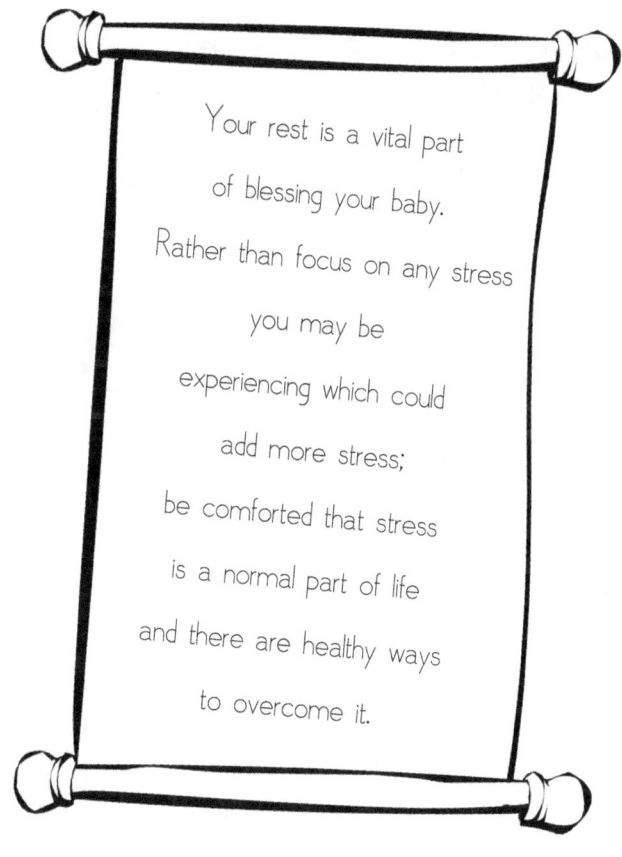

Your rest is a vital part of blessing your baby. Rather than focus on any stress you may be experiencing which could add more stress; be comforted that stress is a normal part of life and there are healthy ways to overcome it.

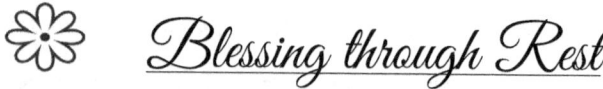

# Blessing through Rest

1- Take time to rest and get rid of tension whenever you can. Sit down, put your feet up, and take deep, relaxed breaths.

2- Do something to help someone else; demonstrating compassion, benevolence and kindness towards another helps you!

3- Watch a comedy or listen to a comedian. Laughter is a great stress reliever.

4- Listen to soothing music or sounds of nature.

5- Have someone rub your back, hands and feet.

6- Exercise.

7- Pray.

8- Forgive others; bless them instead.

9- Smile. Smiling has been shown to reduce stress and release a general feeling of well-being.

10-Use essential oils to help reduce stress. Put your favorite scents in a diffuser, or mix a few drops with some coconut oil and have someone give you a massage with it.

# Chapter 5

# Eating

"There is nothing better for a person than that he should
eat and drink and find enjoyment in his toil. This also,
I saw, is from the hand of God, for apart from him
who can eat, or who can have enjoyment?"
Ecclesiastes 2:24-25

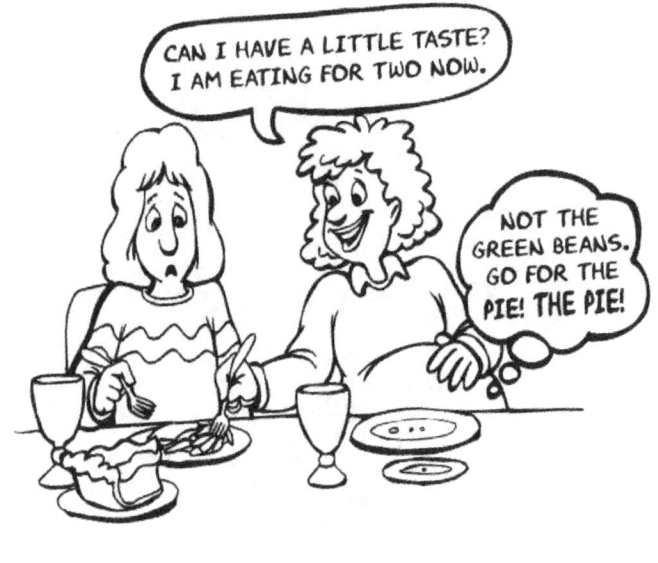

You most likely already know you should be eating a variety of whole foods in their most natural state possible and drinking LOTS of water. Also, presumably, you are taking prenatal vitamins and/or whole food supplements and maintaining a well balanced diet. So, here are some fun facts about what you eat and how it effects your baby in ways you may not ever have heard about.

The food flavors of what you eat do cross the placenta into your amniotic fluid so your baby will taste whatever you've just eaten and acquire a taste for all the foods you like to eat. The baby's taste buds actually form in the womb from about 15 weeks onwards and are fully formed around week 30.

Babies don't actually need to eat or drink as they're fed through the umbilical cord, so if your baby chooses to drink amniotic fluid, its because it likes the taste! This continues even when your baby is breast feeding, as traces of your last meal will flavor your breast milk and baby will actually prefer the flavors that are most familiar from in vitro.

> Nothing would be more tiresome
> than eating and drinking
> if God had not made them a pleasure
> as well as a necessity.
>
> ~Voltaire

Your baby actually seems to savor some meals. After you've eaten something sugary, baby is most likely to sip the fluid more quickly. Foods that have a strong flavor (such as curry and garlic), give the amniotic fluid a stronger taste that might even make baby grimace. If you drink a strong cup of coffee, its heart rate will quicken.

Dr. Benoist Schaal, researcher at the Dijon-Dresden European Laboratory for Taste and Smell (Centre National de la Recherche Scientifique), states that eating habits start in the womb. The scientists asked a group of pregnant women to consume anise flavored cookies. Once the moms gave birth, researchers tested their kids along with others whose mothers hadn't consumed the cookies. They found that the former recognized the smell and showed a good disposition towards it, while the latter rejected it. Some research suggests that if you associate the taste of something with pleasure, so will your baby.

One sweet treat in particular has been proven to benefit your baby! Recent research has found that eating chocolate during pregnancy not only appeals to your unborn baby, but will also make him/her happier and less irritable in the first few years of life. One study showed that the more chocolate a woman ate during pregnancy, the more likely her baby was likely to laugh, smile, not show fear and be soothed more easily. (15) That is great news for chocolate-lovers!

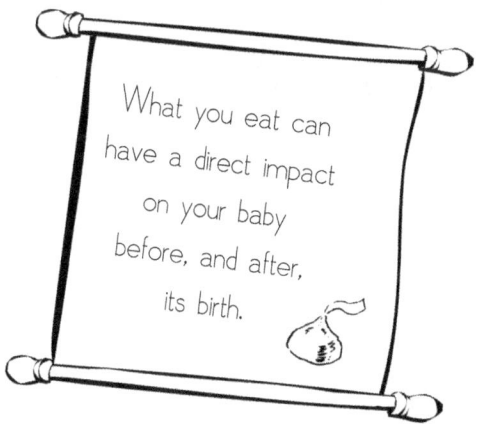

What you eat can
have a direct impact
on your baby
before, and after,
its birth.

# ❁ *Blessing through Eating*

1- Eat a well balanced diet. Consume lots of leafy greens. Eat foods in as close to their natural state as possible.

2- Drink lots of water. 8-10 glasses per day.

3- Avoid soda, caffeine and non-nutritional food items.

4- Eat dark chocolate. Darker is healthier. Organic is best.

5- Take antioxidant supplements and quality prenatal vitamins.

6- Supplement with probiotic foods like kefir, kombucha, yogurt, kimchi, saurkraut, etc..

# Chapter 6

# Exercising

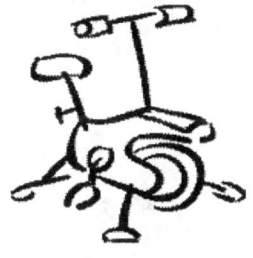

"Do you not know that those who run in a race all run,
but only one receives the prize? Run in such a way that
you may win. Everyone who competes in the games
exercises self-control in all things."
1 Corinthians 9:24-25a

"Physical fitness can neither be achieved
by wishful thinking nor outright purchase."

....................

~Joseph Pilates

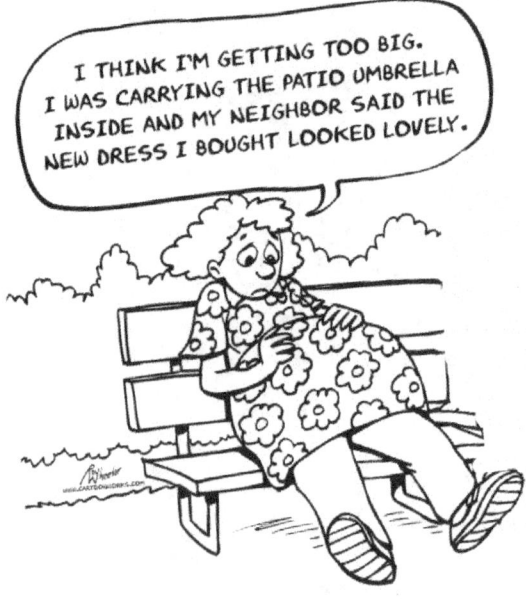

*Healthy Moms typically, gain an average of 25-35 lbs. during
their pregnancy. This is beneficial for baby, when it is done wisely.

Make healthy eating choices and exercise a lifelong habit!

According to medical experts, when the pregnant mom exercises it is good for both mother and child. The baby reaps many benefits, also.

## 7 Ways Your Baby Benefits from Your Exercise Routine:

**1. Heart Health.** One study found that when an expectant mother works out, her baby gleans cardiac benefits in the form of lower fetal heart rates.

**2. Mature Lungs.** Babies of women who exercised had a more mature respiratory system, suggesting they would fare better after birth.

**3. Less likely to be obese.** Babies born to moms who didn't exercise had higher-than-average weights. "The modest reduction in birth weight may lead to a long-term reduction in the risk for obesity in off-spring of women who exercised in pregnancy," says Dr. Paul L. Hofman of the University of Auckland.

**4. Increased I.Q.** Babies born of exercising women do better on standardized intelligence, general intelligence, and oral language tests at one year of age and after.

**5. Overall Health.** Infants of exercising women do significantly better on the Bayley Scales of Infant Development (BSID), which are used to diagnose infants for cognitive, motor, and behavioral development. Even five years after birth results held steady!

**6. Less Toxins, better placenta.** Babies of exercising moms receive more nutrients, feel less stress, are given more oxygen, and have a less toxic environment. Placentas of moms who exercise regularly through early and mid pregnancy grow faster and function better. When mom's exercise they increase their blood volume another 10 percent. With more hemoglobin transporting oxygen during exercise, more blood is pumped with each beat of the mom's heart. So the placenta provides more blood and oxygen to the baby than usual.

**7. Better birth experience.** Fewer pre-term baby interventions. Fewer birth complications.

## Follow these exercise tips for safety:

If you haven't exercised for a while, begin with as little as five minutes of physical activity a day. Build up to 10 minutes, then 15 minutes, and so on, until you reach at least 30 minutes a day.

No matter how dedicated you are to being in shape, don't exercise to the point of exhaustion. Stop if you experience dizziness or can't carry on a conversation.

Drink plenty of fluids to stay hydrated, and be careful to avoid overheating.

---

An early-morning walk
is a blessing
for the whole day.

. . . . . . . . . . . . . . . . . .

-Henry David Thoreau

# ❁ *Blessing through Smell*

Yes! When your baby is born, he/she is already imprinted with the odor of his amniotic fluid. This odor imprint helps him find your nipple, which has a similar odor. This smell imprint from its mother, helps the baby derive feelings of calmness and pain reduction from his mom's scent.

Gradually, over the next few days after birth, your baby starts to prefer the odor of your breast and can be comforted with the unique scent of its fluid.

In fact, even two weeks after birth, infants are more attracted to their mother's breast odor than to that of formula. Oxytocin is believed to be the main contributor to this effect.

Similarly, for the mom, high oxytocin causes a mother to become familiar with the unique odor of her newborn infant, and once attracted to it, she prefers her own baby's odor above all others. (34)

---

"Every good thing given and every perfect gift is from above, coming down from the Father of lights, with whom there is no variation or shifting shadow."

James 1:17

---

# ❀ *Blessing through Exercising*

1- Do an aerobic activity 3-4x a week. For most pregnant women, at least 30 minutes of moderate exercise is recommended.

2- Shorter, but more frequent workouts can help you stay in shape, too. For example, divide the 30 minutes up into 3, 10 minute segments.

3- Maintain flexibility through stretching. Remember to stretch before and after each workout. Stretches in the squating position can help the muscles in that area that will be called on during labor.

4- Walk briskly, swim, row, take the stairs, ride a stationary bike riding, ..

5- Strength training is OK, too, as long as you avoid lifting heavy weights.

6- Put fun music on and dance.

*Remember to consult with your healthcare provider about your exercise.

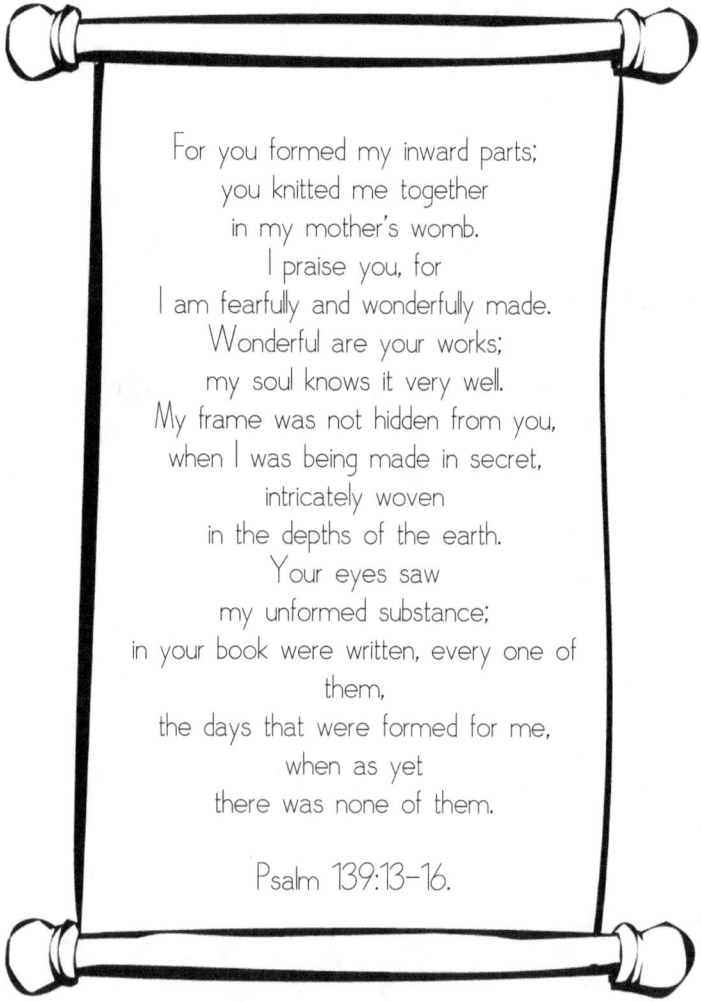

For you formed my inward parts;
you knitted me together
in my mother's womb.
I praise you, for
I am fearfully and wonderfully made.
Wonderful are your works;
my soul knows it very well.
My frame was not hidden from you,
when I was being made in secret,
intricately woven
in the depths of the earth.
Your eyes saw
my unformed substance;
in your book were written, every one of
them,
the days that were formed for me,
when as yet
there was none of them.

Psalm 139:13-16.

# Beautiful Blessings

"The Lord bless you and keep you;
the Lord make his face to shine upon you
and be gracious to you; the Lord lift up
his countenance upon you and give you peace."
Numbers 6: 24-26

"As a mother,
my job is to take care
of what is possible
and trust God
with the impossible."

..........................

-Ruth Bell Graham

# A Family Blessing

"The Blessing," by Gary Smalley and John Trent.

1- A meaningful touch. Isaac kissed Jacob before he blessed him and Jacob put his hands on his son's head as he blessed them.

2- A spoken message. Words are powerful and should be treated as such. Well thought out and prayed over words should be spoken in a blessing.

3- Attach high value to the one being blessed. A blessing has honor attached to it. To honor is to draw from within and bestow on another.

4- Picturing a special future for the one being blessed. All the promises of God are yea and amen in Christ. We have a blessed hope in this life and in the life to come.

5- An active commitment to the one being blessed. Job was a man who blessed his children and even after they were grown he offered sacrifices and prayers on their behalf in case any of them had sinned in their hearts against the Lord. Job 1:5. (33)

# Sixteen Things to Pray for Your Children.

Tom Harmon Ministries/ tdharmon.com

1- Their salvation.

2- Their mate.

3- That they would fall in love with God's Word.

4- That God would keep them from the evil one.

5- That they would have a conscience void of offence before God and man.

6- That their character would be more valuable to them than their credentials.

7- That they would stand up for what is right even if it means standing alone.

8- That they would be kept from the love of money.

9- That they would be kept morally pure.

10- That they would have the heart of a servant.

11- That eternity would burn in their hearts.

12- That sin would always be distasteful to them and that they would be broken easily over sin.

13- That they would love each other.

14- That they would trust God with their parents and not allow rebellion to set in.

15- Regardless the hardship, that they may never become bitter against God.

16- That our boys would be glad to be boys and our girls glad to be girls. (32)

## *A Personal Prayer for My Baby* –

_____

_____

_____

_____

_____

_____

_____

*Train up a child
in the way he should go;
even when he is old
he will not depart from it.*

*Proverbs 22:6*

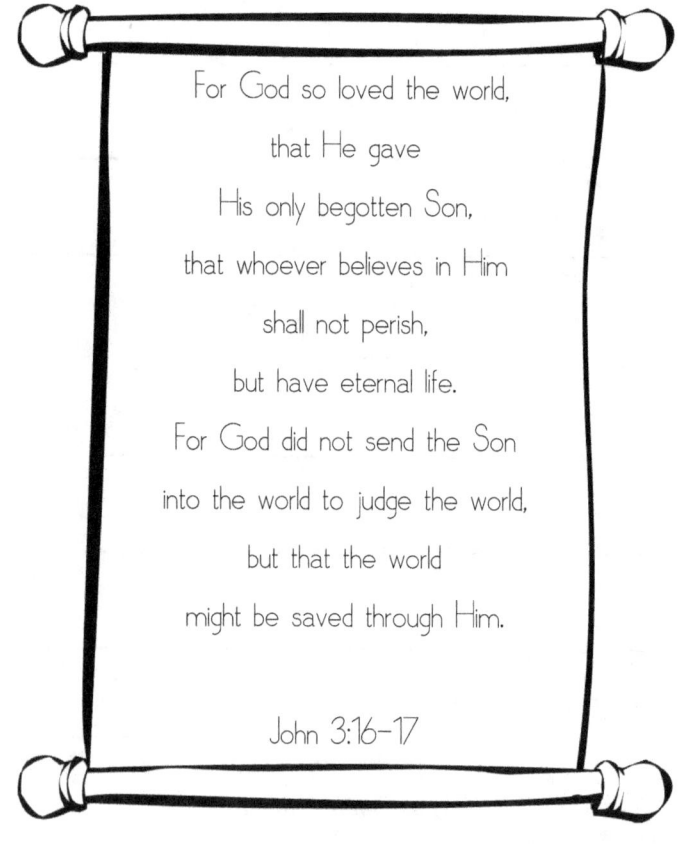

For God so loved the world,
that He gave
His only begotten Son,
that whoever believes in Him
shall not perish,
but have eternal life.
For God did not send the Son
into the world to judge the world,
but that the world
might be saved through Him.

John 3:16-17

# References

....be admonished by these: of making many books there is
no end; and much study is a weariness of the flesh.

Ecclesiastes 12:12

(1) The New York Times, "The Experience of Touch: Research Points to a Critical Role." By Daniel Goleman February 02, 1988

(2) Science Daily, "Rockabye Baby: Research Shows Gentle Singing Soothes Sick Infants." ScienceDaily (Feb. 13, 2006)

(3) "Praying Through Your Pregnancy: An Inspirational Week-by-Week Guide for Bonding with Your Baby," by Jennifer Polimino, March 28, 2010

(4-8) Psychology Today, September/October 1998, Volume 31, No. 5, Pages 44-48, 78, By Janet L. Hopson

(9) How the Mother's Emotions Affecct the Baby Before Birth, The Well Baby Book by Mike Samuels, M.D. and Nancy Samuels, pages 49 - 52

(10-13) http://www.welcomebabyhome.com

(14) Babies May Inherit their Mother's Eating Habits in the Womb, Posted on February 22, 2012 by Jaime Menchén in Med-Health

(15) How your diet affects your unborn baby, By Pregnancy & birth, http://www.askamum.co.uk

(16) Pregnancy and exercise: Baby, let's move!, by mayo Clinic Staff, mayoclinic.com

(17-18) Babies' Language Starts In The Womb, Viewzone.com

(19-22) Prenatal Stimulation For A Smart Baby, By Olivia Lim and Safia

(23) actionlife.org

(24) Study: Unborn Babies Can Differentiate Touch, Pain in Womb, by Steven Ertelt, Washington, DC, LifeNews.com ,9/9/11

(25) Scientific American, Baby's Little Smiles: Building a Relationship with Mom, By Yoshiaki Kikuchi and Madoka Noriuchi September 23, 2008

(26) Can Smiling Make You Happy? , Kleinke, C.L., Peterson, T.R., & Rutledge, T.R. (1998). Effects of self-generated facial expressions on mood. Journal of Personality and Social Psychology, 74, 272-279.

(27) Give Your Body a Boost -- With Laughter
Why, for some, laughter is the best medicine
By R. Morgan Griffin, WebMD Feature

(28) Do Good, Feel Good
New research shows that helping others may be the key to happiness., By Lisa Farino for MSN Health & Fitness

(29) Education oasis, Building Baby's Brain: The Role of Music, by Diane Bales, Ph.D.

(30) What Are the Benefits of Classical Music on the Brain?
By Sophie Johnson, eHow Contributor

(31) info@excellenceinwriting.com • 1-800-856-5815
"Music is not "Nice,"" by Andrew Pudewa

"Your Own Prenatal Classroom," by F. Rene Van de Carr, M.D.
Fetal Bill Of Rights.

"Mom's exercise helps fetal lungs mature."
By Janet Raloff.

"Mom's Exercise Helps Baby's Heart," By Dennis Thompson.
http://www.getfitforbirth.com/happier-smarter-babies/

Scripture quotes from the Holy Bible, NASB,KJV,ESV

(32) TDHarmon.com, Tom Harmon Ministries, "16 Things to
Pray for Your Children."

(33) "The Blessing" by Gary Smalley and John Trent.

(34) The Chemistry of Attachment, by Linda F. Palmer, DC,
Reprinted from the API News, Vol. 5, No. 2, 2002

---

Congratulations on your pregnancy.
May you be blessed with continued joy!


Wendy@MyMorningSickness.com

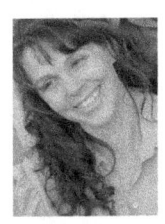

## About the Author

Wendy and her husband, Kevin, with their 10 children, live near Yosemite National Park in California. She created the site: MyMorningSickness.com to help provide information and support for all pregnant Moms.

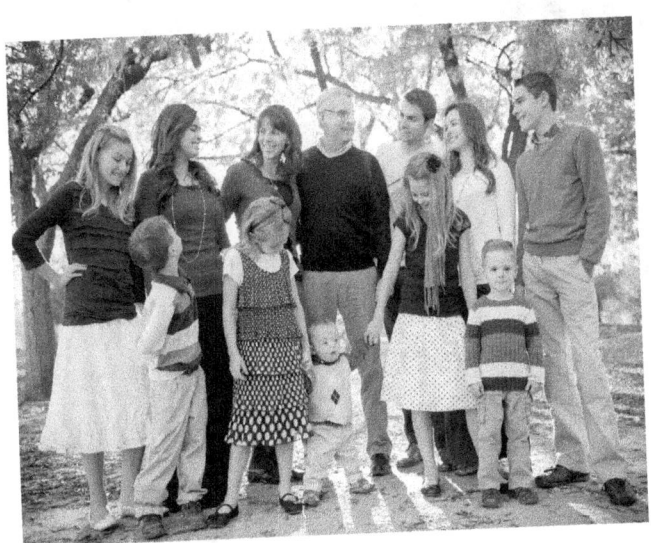

The Shaw Family

Kevin & Wendy, Chase, Holly, Macy, Justus,

Elley, Amy, Lilly, Peter and Daniel & Joshua

Other Books By this Author:

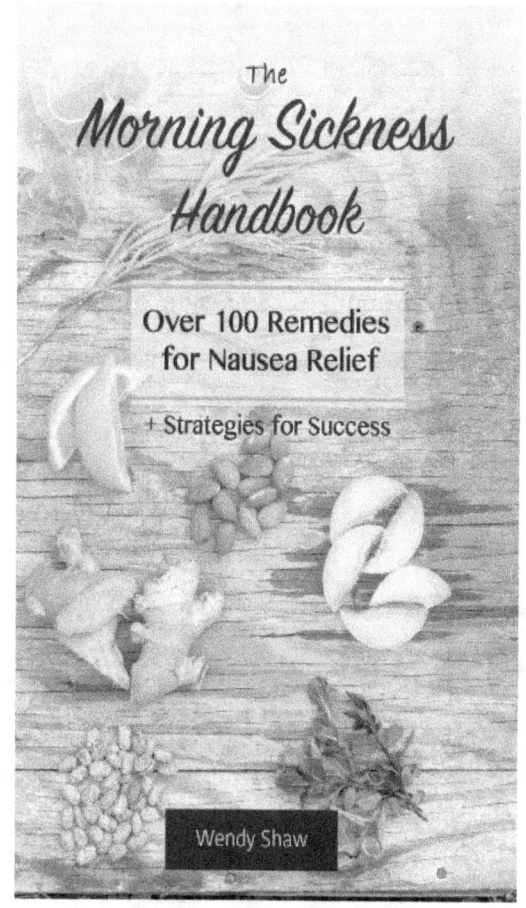

The Morning Sickness Handbook by Wendy Shaw

Order from MyMorningSickness.com or Amazon.com

*" Faith is deliberate confidence in the character of God whose ways you may not understand at the time."*

*-Oswald Chambers*